I0077297

The Patient's Guide

Vertebroplasty and Kyphoplasty

Adam E. M. Eltorai, MD, PhD
Omowunmi Ajibola, MD
Terrance T. Healey, MD

Praeclarus Press, LLC

www.PraeclarusPress.com

Praeclarus Press, LLC
2504 Sweetgum Lane
Amarillo, Texas 79124 USA
806-367-9950
www.PraeclarusPress.com

DISCLAIMER
The information contained in this publication is advisory only and
is not intended to replace sound clinical judgment or individualized
patient care. The author disclaims all warranties, whether expressed
or implied, including any warranty as the quality, accuracy, safety,
or suitability of this information for any particular purpose.

ISBN: 978-1-946665-32-4
©2020 Omowunmi Ajibola. All rights reserved.
Email: omowunmiajibola@gmail.com

Cover Design: Ken Tackett
Developmental Editing: Kathleen Kendall-Tackett
Copy Editing: Chris Tackett
Layout & Design: Nelly Murariu

CONTENTS

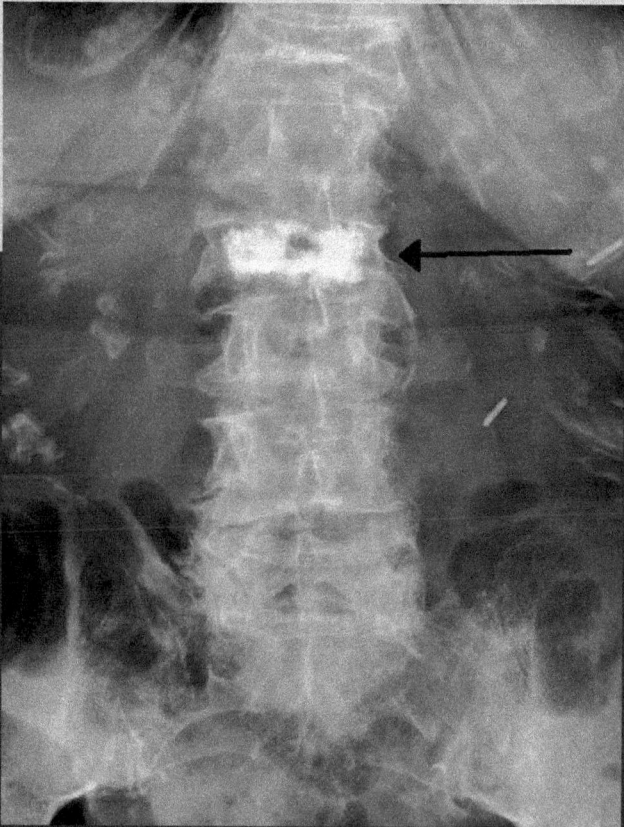

Cement in a vertebra as seen on plain Xray.

WHAT ARE VERTEBROPLASTY AND KYPHOPLASTY?

Vertebroplasty **and** kyphoplasty are image-guided procedures that involves the injection of cement material into a collapsed vertebral body. There are mild differences between vertebroplasty and kyphoplasty: kyphoplasty involves creating a cavity in the vertebral body in which the cement is injected, all done through a percutaneous needle, and is known as a low-pressure injection, while vertebroplasty doesn't involve creating a cavity, thus, cement is injected through a percutaneous needle into the vertebral body known as a high-pressure injection.

WHY ARE VERTEBROPLASTY AND KYPHOPLASTY PERFORMED?

It is usually performed in patients with osteoporosis, usually elderly patients, with recent vertebral body compression fractures who are not good surgical candidates. Some patients may not want to have a long hospital stay and may want this procedure done as patients can be sent home the same day. It is usually done as a treatment or palliative effort for painful compression fractures. Other reasons include treatment for aggressive vertebral hemangiomas and metastatic disease.

HOW DO I PREPARE FOR THE PROCEDURE?

Preparation for the procedure begins from talking to the doctor performing the procedure. The doctor should explain to you what the procedure is, as well as the risks and benefits of doing the procedure. You should let the doctor know what medications you are taking as the doctor needs to know which medications can be taken and which ones need to be stopped before the procedure, and if they do need to be stopped, how long before the procedure to stop the medications. It is also important

It is advised not to have any food after midnight.

to discuss how soon after the procedure the medications can be restarted. Medications such as blood thinners are important to know. You should make sure that you understand the procedure is usually done under some sort of sedation, so you will be advised not to have any food after midnight. Take a bath or shower before the procedure. Avoid using scented lotion or perfumes. Do not wear any jewelry and for those who use contact lenses, do not wear them either.

WHAT KIND OF EQUIPMENT IS USED FOR THE PROCEDURE?

There is much equipment needed for the procedure. A hollow needle or tube called a trochlar is used to anchor the vertebral body and helps as a delivery vehicle to deliver the orthopedic cement. The orthopedic cement usually includes an ingredient called polymethylmethacrylate or PMMA.

A fluoroscopy machine is a machine that uses X-rays to obtain real-time imaging of the vertebral bones. This helps with visualizing the vertebral bone that the procedure is being performed on, as well as with placement of the trochlar needle. Other equipment includes a radiographic table and a monitor to help see the images, as well as equipment to help monitor vital signs such as pulse oximetry and blood pressure machines, as well as IV medications that will be administered.

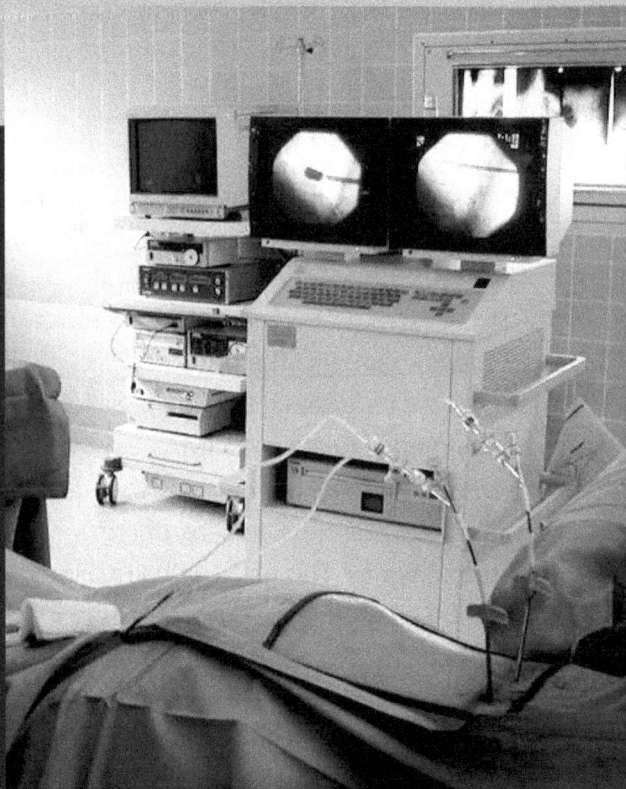

Setup for Kyphoplasty.

HOW IS THE PROCEDURE PERFORMED?

The procedure is usually performed by an interventional radiologist. Sometimes they can be done by orthopedic surgeons and neuroradiologists. If the vertebral body affected is in the thoracic or lumbar spine, you will lay prone (on your stomach), on the table. If it is in the cervical spine, you will be laid supine (on your back). A nurse will insert an IV line into a vein in your hand or arm—this will be used to administer medication and fluids. Sedation medication is given through the IV. You will be connected to monitors to monitor your blood pressure, oxygen level, and heart rate. The area where is the procedure is to be done is cleaned and made sterile with a cleaning solution. Any hair overlying the area is shaved, and the area is draped with surgical drapes. A local anesthetic is given superficially and into the deep tissues. Using fluoroscopy guidance, the trochlar needles are inserted into the vertebral body. If a kyphoplasty is being done, a cavity is made in the vertebral body using a balloon.

If a vertebroplasty is being done, no cavity within the vertebral body is made. Then, cement is injected into the vertebral body under fluoroscopy guidance; it takes about 15-20 minutes for cement to harden.

The trochar needles are then removed. Postprocedural imaging is done to check distribution of the cement. Pressure is held on the skin to prevent bleeding, after which a dry sterile dressing is put on.

WHAT WILL THE PROCEDURE FEEL LIKE?

During the procedure, you should feel no pain due to the combination of local anesthesia and general sedation given. You will be in deep sleep due to the sedation given. If you should feel anything during the procedure, it will be pressure. If you indicate that you are feeling any pain, either more sedation or more local anesthesia is given.

WHAT HAPPENS AFTER THE PROCEDURE?

After the procedure, you are moved to the recovery unit and monitored for a period of time, depending on the preferences of the doctor performing the procedure. This is to make sure you tolerated the procedure well and have no acute symptoms such as shortness of breath, hematoma, or back pain. During this time, the interventional radiologist will have a discussion with you and your family/loved ones as to how the procedure went and whether it was a technical success or not.

Afterward, you will be sent home, usually the same day. Sometimes you may stay overnight for observation and sent home the next day. Some restrictions will be placed on you, such as limiting strenuous activities like heaving lifting. After a few days, you should be able to resume normal activities.

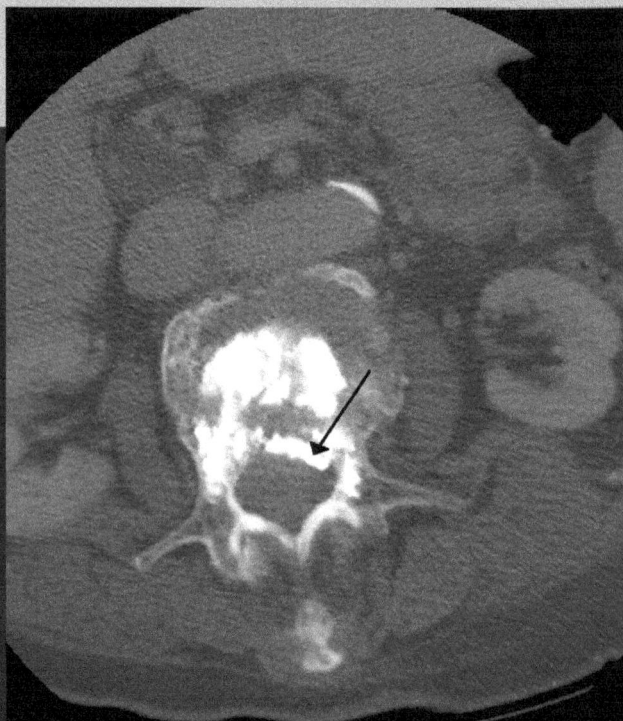

A CT image of cement used in kyphoplasty that has entered the spinal channel and is pressing on the spinal cord resulting in neurological symptoms.

WHAT ARE THE RESULTS OF THE PROCEDURE?

As mentioned above, soon after the procedure is done while recovering, the interventional radiologist will discuss the procedure with you and whether it was a technical success or not. Within a few days, you should feel minimal to no back pain. You should be able to resume normal daily activities.

WHAT ARE THE BENEFITS OF THE PROCEDURE? WHAT ARE THE RISKS OF THE PROCEDURE?

Benefits of the procedure are as follows:

✓ **No large incision and scar:** The procedure is done through a small incision. If you are having multiple vertebral bodies done, then you will have a few small incisions in your skin rather than a long incision and scar.

✓ **Short recovery time**: Many patients feel relief from their back pain and are able to resume daily activities the same day as the procedure was done. Most patients feel relief and are able to resume daily activities within a few days.

✓ **Short hospital stay:** Vertebroplasty and kyphoplasty are same-day procedures, and patients are usually sent home the same day or the day after the procedure was done.

Risks of the procedure are as follows:

⚠ **Infection and bleeding:** Any procedure where the skin is penetrated carries a risk of infection and bleeding. The risk is small, usually less than 1 in 1000.

⚠ **Leakage of cement:** There is a small change that cement may leak outside of the vertebral body, either into the surrounding soft tissue or into blood vessels. This is why the procedure is done under live fluoroscopy and as soon as any cement is seen leaking, the injection of cement into that vertebral body is stopped.

⚠ Some rare complications from the procedure include worsened back pain and neurological symptoms, such as tingling or paresthesias.

You, the patient, should ensure that the risks and benefits, as well as alternatives of the procedure, are discussed with you and that you understand them before signing the consent.

WHAT ARE THE LIMITATIONS OF VERTEBROPLASTY AND KYPHOPLASTY?

There are a few limitations to the procedure. You should make sure these are discussed with you by the doctor who is going to perform the procedure. Limitations are as follows:

- **Incomplete relief of symptoms**: For a few patients, their symptoms, such as back pain, may not resolve. In some situations, they may even get worse.

- **This procedure will not restore complete vertebral body height:** Basically, your vertebral body cannot go back to the way it was before your injury.

- Long-term, there is a possibility of compression fracture of the vertebral bone the procedure was performed on, as well as adjacent vertebral bones.

FREQUENTLY ASKED QUESTIONS

Does it involve any radiation?

Yes, it does. Radiation use is limited and only when necessary during the procedure.

How long does the procedure take?

That depends on how many vertebral bones are being worked on. Most times, the procedure itself takes about 45 mins to an hour. But between sedation and positioning, it takes usually about an hour and half to two hours.

What is the follow-up like?

In most cases, no follow-up is needed. If you start having back pain again or notice back pain that is progressing, you should schedule a visit with your doctor. Most commonly, a CT scan of the back, thoracic, or lumbar depending on where the pain is and where the procedure as done is done to evaluate the bones.

GLOSSARY

OSTEOPOROSIS

A medical condition in which bones become weak and brittle.

HEMANGIOMAS

Noncancerous growth of blood vessels that can occur anywhere in the body, most commonly occurs in the vertebral bones and skin.

OSSEOUS METASTATIC DISEASE

Bony spread of cancer. It can be very painful.

INTERVENTIONAL RADIOLOGIST

A medical doctor who is trained in performing minimally invasive procedures using imaging techniques, such as X-rays and CTs.

NPO

A Latin word nil per os, which means nothing by mouth. Before many procedures requiring sedation, patients are usually required to be NPO for a certain time.

CEMENT

The material injected into the vertebral bone. PMMA or polymethylmethacrylate is the active ingredient and is a type of glass. It is not the same type of cement used in construction.

VERTEBRAL BONE/BODY

Bone that make up the spine. They are load-bearing bones that can undergo compression when the load is too much for them to bear.

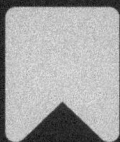

ADDITIONAL RESOURCES

MY CONTACTS

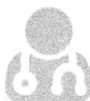

NAME

CONTACT

NAME

CONTACT

NAME

CONTACT

NAME

CONTACT

MY APPOINTMENTS

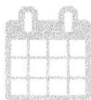

MONDAY

Date:
_____

THURSDAY

Date:
_____

TUESDAY

Date:
_____

FRIDAY

Date:
_____

WEDNESDAY

Date:
_____

SATURDAY

Date:
_____

MY QUESTIONS

MY QUESTIONS

MY QUESTIONS

MY QUESTIONS

MY QUESTIONS

MY NOTES

MY NOTES

MY NOTES

MY NOTES

MY NOTES

MY NOTES